ISBN: 9781073638079

7-DAY DIET
For Women

Gail Johnson, M.S.

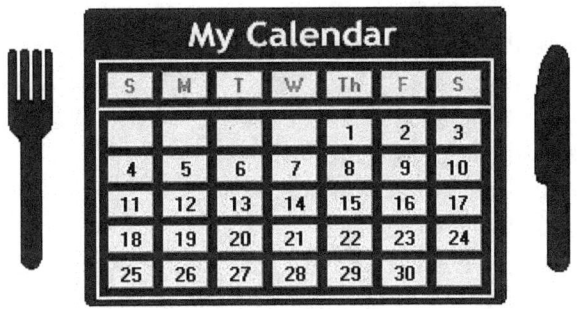

NoPaperPress™

Note: At publication, the off-the-shelf foods used in some of this book were widely available in most supermarkets. But food products come and go. So if there is a frozen entrée or soup selection in this diet that is out of stock, or that's been discontinued, or perhaps you don't like, or that you forgot to pick up while shopping, please substitute another food that has **approximately** the same caloric value and nutritional content. In this regard, many dieters have found the foods listed in the Appendices at the end of this book to be very helpful.

CONTENTS

When to Use the 7-Day Diet

If you're in weight maintenance mode but notice your weight creeping up. You want to stop the upward trend and lose a few pounds as well. Here's the perfect solution: Use the *7-Day Diet* to quickly lose those unwanted few kilos!

You've let your weight get out of control. So you decide to go on a diet. It doesn't matter what diet, or how much weight you want to lose. Your first move should be to go on the *7-Day Diet* lose a quick 3 to 4 lbs and get on the right track. After the 7-day diet does its job you can switch to a longer-term diet. My suggestion would be either the 30-Day Quick Diet or the 90-Day Smart Diet, both eBooks published by NoPaperPress.

Additionally, before you begin any weight loss program you need to make sure your health will allow you to lower your caloric intake and increase your physical activity. A medical checkup is in order which may be as simple as a visit to a physician who is familiar with your medical history, or it may be a thorough physical exam. The physician conducting the medical exam should be made aware of and should approve the specific weight loss diet you're planning

What's in this eBook?

This eBook actually contains two 7-day diets: a 1200 Calorie diet, and for even faster weight loss a 900 Calorie diet. Both diets have a meal plan (menu) for each and every day. And every day features a "Recipe and Diet Tip of the Day."

Which Calorie Level is for You?

900 Calorie Diet: Smaller women, older women and inactive women should consider the 900 Calorie diet.
1200 Calorie Diet: Larger women, younger women and active women should choose the 1200 Calorie diet.

Note: Due to the very low calorie level, the 900-Calorie diet may not quite provide the protein, carbs, fat, vitamins, minerals and fiber you need for good health. Since it's a short term (7-Day) diet, however, this should not be a problem for most healthy people. If you have any health problems or concerns, you definitely should avoid the 900-Calorie diet. Additionally, because nearly everyone feels hungry on 900 Calorie per day, this is not an easy diet to stay with.

How Much Weight Will You Lose?

Weight loss occurs when your food energy intake is less than the total energy you expend. This difference in calories is referred to as your calorie deficit. How much weight you lose depends on the magnitude of your calorie deficit. Physiologists have long known that to lose one kg requires a deficit of approximately 7700 kcal. Therefore, if a person's total calorie deficit over time is known, their weight loss over time can be calculated.

On the 7-Day Diet, **most women lose 3 to 4 pounds** – depending on whether they select the 1200 or 900 Calorie diet. Smaller women, older women and less active women will lose a bit less and larger women, younger women and more active women often lose much more. Exactly how much weight you will lose depends on how much you weigh, your age and your activity level. For the full story see *Weight Control - U.S. Edition* by Vincent Antonetti, PhD - also published by NoPaperPress.

How to Use This eBook

First, depending on your size, your age and how active you are, choose the diet calorie level that's right for you, either 900 or 1,200 kcal per day.
- For the 900-Caloriel Diet go to page 8.
- For the 1200-Calorie Diet go to page 16.
- For Shopping Tips go to **Appendix A** page 33.

900 Calorie Daily Menus

Day 1 – 900 Calorie Meal Plan

BREAKFAST	Kcal	Totals
Orange juice (½ cup)	50	
Wheaties (¾ cup) + ½ cup skim milk + ½ banana	190	
Coffee (See **Notes** - page 39)	10	250 Cal
SNACK		
Coffee or tea	10	10 Cal
LUNCH		
Soup (Appendix C - page 42)	140	
Turkey breast (1 oz) on 1 slice rye bread	115	
Pickle spear	0	
Lettuce & tomato slices	20	
Water	0	275 Cal
SNACK		
Coffee or tea	10	10 Cal
DINNER		
Baked salmon with salsa (**Day 1 Recipe** - page 25)	215	
Summer squash, zucchini and tomatoes	60	
Large tossed green salad (1½ Tbsp low-cal dressing)*	70	
Water	0	345 Cal
* See page 38.		
SNACK		
Coffee or tea	10	10 Cal
		900 Cal

Day 2 – 900 Calorie Meal Plan

BREAKFAST	kcal	Totals
Orange juice (½ cup)	50	
Soft-boiled egg	80	
Whole-grain toast (1 slice) (See **Notes** - page 39)	65	
Coffee	10	205 Cal
SNACK		
Coffee or tea	10	10 Cal
LUNCH		
Salad (3 oz tuna, 1 tsp Evoo, onions & celery)	175	
Lettuce & tomato wedges	20	
Rye bread (1 slice)	65	
Diet soda or water	0	290 Cal
SNACK		
Coffee or tea	10	10 Cal
DINNER		
Veggie burger – (1 patty) (Day 2 Recipe - page 26)	100	
Seeded hamburger roll	140	
Large tossed green salad with 1½ Tbsp low-cal	70	
Fresh fruit in season (apple, peach, etc)	70	
Water	0	380 Cal
SNACK		
Coffee or tea	10	10 Cal
		905 Cal

Day 3 – 900 Calorie Meal Plan

BREAKFAST	kcal	Totals
Cantaloupe (½ medium)	50	
Wild blueberry pancakes (Day 3 Recipe - page 27)	190	
Light syrup (1 Tbsp)	30	
Coffee	10	280 Cal
SNACK		
Coffee or tea	10	10 Cal
LUNCH		
Peanut butter (1 Tbsp) on 1 slice whole-grain bread	170	
Skim milk (6 oz)	70	
Fresh fruit in season (peach, pear, etc)	70	310 Cal
SNACK		
Coffee or tea	10	10 Cal
DINNER		
Broiled veal chop (4 oz lean)	200	
Large tossed green salad (1½ Tbsp low-cal dressing)	70	
Hot or iced tea	10	280 Cal
SNACK		
Coffee or tea	10	10 Cal
		900 Cal

Day 4 – 900 Calorie Meal Plan

BREAKFAST	kcal	Totals
Fresh sliced orange	75	
Cheerios (1 cup) + ½ cup skim milk	160	
Coffee	10	245 Cal
SNACK		
Coffee or tea	10	10 Cal
LUNCH		
Cottage cheese (1 cup low fat)	180	
Large tossed green salad with 1½ Tbsp low-cal	70	
Water	0	250 Cal
SNACK		
Handful unsalted mixed nuts	100	100 Cal
DINNER		
Grilled chicken sausage (2 links about 2½ oz per link)	180	
Green beans - steamed	25	
Fresh fruit in season (apple, pear, etc)	70	
Hot or iced tea	10	285 Cal
SNACK		
Coffee or tea	10	10 Cal
		890 Cal

12

Day 5 – 900 Calorie Meal Plan

BREAKFAST	kcal	Totals
Orange juice (½ cup)	50	
Wheaties (¾ cup) + ½ cup skim milk + ½ banana	190	
Coffee	10	250 Cal
SNACK		
Coffee or tea	10	10 Cal
LUNCH		
Grilled Swiss cheese sandwich (2 oz low-fat cheese)	310	
Pickle spear	0	
Hot or iced tea	10	320 Cal
SNACK		
Coffee or tea	10	10 Cal
DINNER		
Frozen chicken entree (Day 5 Recipe - page 29)	220	
Large tossed green salad with 1½ Tbsp low-cal	70	
Hot or iced tea	10	300 Cal
SNACK		
Coffee or tea	10	10 Cal
		900 Cal

Day 6 – 900 Calorie Meal Plan

BREAKFAST	kcal	Totals
Orange juice (½ cup)	20	
Scrambled egg (Notes - page 40)	80	
Whole-grain toast (1 slice)	65	
Coffee	10	205 Cal
SNACK		
Coffee or tea	10	10 Cal
LUNCH		
Subway 6" (Ham, Cheese +veggies)*	260	
Hot or iced tea	10	270 Cal
SNACK		
Yogurt (6 oz, nonfat, any flavor)	90	90 Cal
DINNER		
Baked Herb-Crusted Cod (Day 6 Recipe - page 31)	230	
Asparagus (7 spears cooked & drained)	20	
Fresh fruit in season (apple, plum, etc)	70	
Water		320 Cal
SNACK		
Coffee or tea	10	10 Cal
		905 Cal

Day 7 – 900 Calorie Meal Plan

BREAKFAST	kcal	Totals
Orange juice (½ cup)	50	
Shredded Wheat (1 cup) + ½ cup skim milk + 10 raisins	230	
Coffee	10	290 Cal
SNACK		
Coffee or tea	10	10 Cal
LUNCH		
Turkey frank (2 oz) with mustard & relish	150	
Hot dog bun (½)	65	
Diet soda		215 Cal
SNACK		
Coffee or tea	10	10 Cal
DINNER		
Pasta with Marinara sauce (Day 7 Recipe - page 32)	225	
Large tossed green salad with 1½ Tbsp low-cal	70	
Fresh fruit in season (peach, plum, etc)	70	
Water	0	365 Cal
SNACK		
Coffee or tea	10	10 Cal
		900 Cal

1200 Calorie Daily Menus

Day 1 – 1200 Calorie Meal Plan

BREAKFAST	kcal	Totals
Cantaloupe (½ medium)	50	
Wheaties (¾ cup) + ½ cup skim milk + ½ banana	190	
Coffee (Notes - page 39)	10	250 Cal
SNACK		
Coffee or tea	10	10 Cal
LUNCH		
Soup (Appendix C - page 42)	140	
Turkey breast (1 oz) on 1 slice rye bread (½	115	
Pickle spear	0	
Lettuce & tomato slices	20	
Hot or iced tea	10	285 Cal
SNACK		
Coffee or tea	10	10 Cal
DINNER		
Baked salmon with salsa (Day 1 Recipe - page 25)	215	
Summer squash, zucchini and tomatoes	60	
Brown rice (½ cup)	100	
Large tossed green salad (1½ Tbsp low-cal dressing)*	70	
Fresh fruit in season (apple, peach, etc)	70	
Water	0	515 Cal
* See page 38.		
SNACK		
Fiber One Chocolate Fudge Brownie	90	
Skim milk (4 oz)	40	130 Cal
		1200 Cal

Day 2 – 1200 Calorie Meal Plan

BREAKFAST	kcal	Totals
Orange juice (½ cup)	50	
Soft-boiled egg (or poached)	80	
Whole-grain toast (1 slice) (Notes - page 40)	65	
Coffee	10	205 Cal
SNACK		
Coffee or tea	10	10 Cal
LUNCH		
Salad (3 oz tuna, 1 tsp Evoo, onions & celery)	175	
Lettuce & tomato wedges	20	
Rye bread (1 slice)	65	
Fresh fruit in season (apple, plum, etc)	70	
Coffee or tea	10	340 Cal
SNACK		
Yogurt (6 oz, nonfat, any flavor)*	90	
Coffee or tea	10	100 Cal
DINNER		
Veggie burger – (1 patty) (Day 2 Recipe - page 26)	100	
Low-fat cheddar cheese (1 thin slice)	50	
Seeded hamburger roll	140	
Large tossed green salad with 1½ Tbsp low-cal	70	
Beets (3 small)	45	
Hot or iced tea	10	415 Cal
SNACK		
Graham Cracker (2 squares)	60	
Skim milk (6 oz)	60	120 Cal
* Such as Dannon Lite & Fit. (Buy 32 oz & use 6 oz.)		1190 Cal

Day 3 – 1200 Calorie Meal Plan

BREAKFAST	kcal	Totals
Orange juice (½ cup)	50	
Wild blueberry pancakes (Day 3 Recipe - page 27)	190	
Light syrup (2 Tbsp)	60	
Coffee	10	310 Cal
SNACK		
Coffee or tea	10	10 Cal
LUNCH		
Peanut butter (2 Tbsp) on 2 slices whole-grain bread	330	
Skim milk (6 oz)	70	
Fresh fruit in season (peach, plum, etc)	70	470 Cal
SNACK		
Coffee or tea	10	10 Cal
DINNER		
Vegetable bouillon	0	
Broiled pork chop (about ½" thick & trimmed of fat)	260	
Green peas (½ cup)	55	
Large tossed green salad with 1½ Tbsp low-cal	70	
Water with lemon section	15	400 Cal
SNACK		
Coffee or tea	10	10 Cal
		1210 Cal

Day 4 – 1200 Calorie Meal Plan

BREAKFAST	kcal	Totals
Fresh sliced orange	75	
Cheerios (1 cup) + ½ cup skim milk + about 15 raisins*	190	
Coffee	10	275 Cal
SNACK		
Fresh fruit in season (apple, plum, etc)	70	
Coffee or tea	10	80 Cal
LUNCH		
Cottage cheese (1 cup low fat)	180	
Large tossed green salad (1½ Tbsp low-cal dressing)	70	
Small whole-grain roll	80	
Hot or iced tea	10	340 Cal
SNACK		
Handful unsalted mixed nuts	100	
Coffee or tea	10	110 Cal
DINNER		
London Broil (Day 4 Recipe - page 28)	320	
Large tossed green salad with 1½ Tbsp low-cal	70	
Water	0	390 Cal
SNACK		
Coffee or tea	10	10 Cal
* You may substitute 2 blueberries for each raisin.		1205 Cal

Day 5 – 1200 Calorie Meal Plan

BREAKFAST	kcal	Totals
Cantaloupe (½ medium)	50	
Scrambled egg (Notes - page 40)	80	
Whole-grain toast (1 slice)	65	
Coffee	10	205 Cal
SNACK		
Yogurt (6 oz, nonfat, any flavor)	90	
Coffee or tea	10	100 Cal
LUNCH		
Subway 6" (Ham, Cheese +veggies)*	260	
Hot or iced tea	10	270 Cal
SNACK		
Coffee or tea	10	10 Cal
DINNER		
Frozen Entree (Day 5 Recipe - page 29)	300	
Large tossed green salad with 1½ Tbsp low-cal	70	
Fresh fruit in season (peach, plum, etc)	70	
Water with lemon section	15	455 Cal
SNACK		
Two small cookies	150	
Coffee or tea	10	160 Cal
		1200 Cal

Day 6 – 1200 Calorie Meal Plan

BREAKFAST	kcal	Totals
Orange juice (½ cup)	50	
Fried egg	80	
Whole-grain toast (1 slice)	65	
Coffee	10	205 Cal
SNACK		
Yogurt (6 oz, nonfat, any flavor)	90	
Coffee or tea	10	100 Cal
LUNCH		
Grilled Swiss cheese sandwich (2 oz low-fat cheese)	310	
Pickle spear	0	
Hot or iced tea	10	320 Cal
SNACK		
Fresh fruit in season (apple, plum, etc)	70	
Coffee or tea	10	80 Cal
DINNER		
Baked Herb-Crusted Cod (Day 6 Recipe - page 31)	230	
Asparagus (7 spears cooked & drained)	20	
Large tossed green salad with 1½ Tbsp low-cal	70	
Water with lemon section	15	335 Cal
SNACK		
Dark chocolate (1 oz)	150	
Coffee or tea	10	160 Cal
		1200 Cal

Day 7 – 1200 Calorie Meal Plan

BREAKFAST	kcal	Totals
Orange juice (½ cup)	50	
Shredded Wheat (1 cup) + ½ cup skim milk + ½ banana	260	
Coffee	10	320 Cal
SNACK		
Coffee or tea	10	10 Cal
LUNCH		
Turkey frank (2 oz) with mustard & relish	150	
Hot-dog bun	130	
Gelatin dessert (unsweetened)	10	
Diet soda	0	290 Cal
SNACK		
Yogurt (6 oz, nonfat, any flavor)	90	
Coffee or tea	10	100 Cal
DINNER		
Pasta with Marinara sauce (Day 7 Recipe - page 32)	225	
Large tossed green salad with 1½ Tbsp low-cal	70	
Fresh fruit in season (pear, plum, etc)	70	
Italian or French bread (1 slice)	80	
Water with lemon section	15	460 Cal
SNACK		
Coffee or tea	10	10 Cal
		1190 Cal

Recipes & Diet Tips

Day 1 Recipe

Baked Salmon with Salsa

This is a simple, straight-forward recipe. The advantage of a simple recipe is that there are no hidden calories.

    4 - 5 oz salmon fillets

    6 - Tbsp bottled tomato-pepper salsa

Brown salmon fillets in non-stick pan and place in baking dish. Put fillets in an oven preheated to 350 °F for about 10 minutes. Plate the salmon. Stir prepared tomato-pepper salsa and spoon it over the salmon.

Serves 4. One salmon fillet is about 215 Calories.

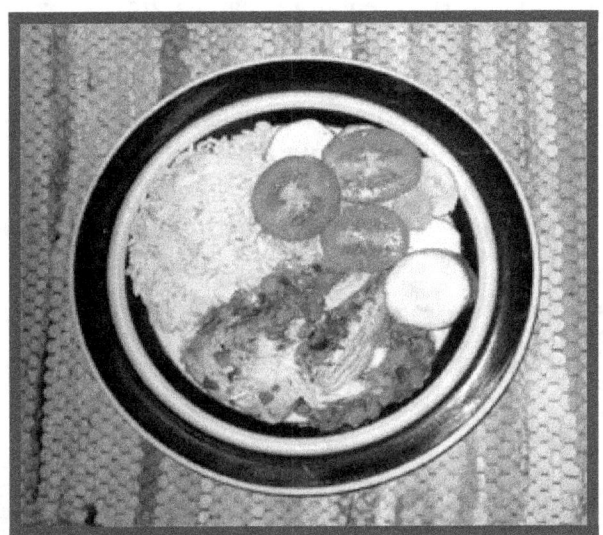

Diet Tip of the Day: **Have soup more often.** Most <u>non-cream-based</u> soups are filling and low-calorie.

Day 2 Recipe

Veggie Burger

Vegetable-based burgers can be purchased at your local supermarket. The patty of a veggie burger can be made from vegetables, soy, nuts, mushrooms, textured vegetable protein, dairy, or a combination of these foods.

Two popular veggie burgers are the Boca Burger and Gardenburger. The Boca Burger is made chiefly from soy protein and wheat gluten. (Boca Burger patties are 2.5 oz each and range from 60 to 90 Calories.) The original Gardenburger is made from mushrooms, onions, brown rice, rolled oats, cheese, and spices. (Gardenburger patties are 2.5 oz each and about 100 Calories.)

To prepare, follow package directions. The version shown below has an added slice of low-fat cheddar cheese. The lettuce, tomato and ketchup shown actually add very few extra calories.

The veggie burger patty plus low-fat cheese amounts to approximately 150 Calories. Add a seeded roll and the total rises to 290 Calories.

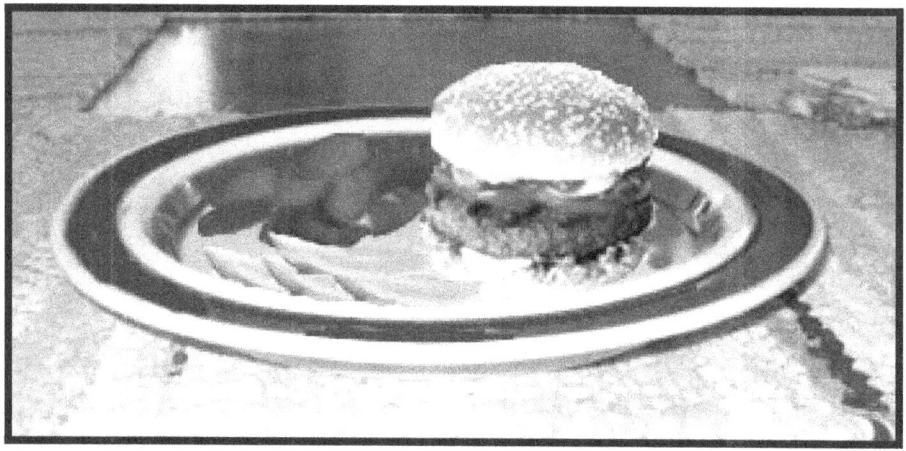

Diet Tip of the Day: **Drink lots of water** – about 8 glasses per day. Add a slice of lemon to make it more interesting. Often, when you think you're hungry, you are just thirsty. So, next time you head for a snack, drink some water first and see if that does it for you.

Day 3 Recipe

Wild-Blueberry Pancakes

This recipe makes a relatively low calorie, wholesome batch of delicious wild blueberry-whole wheat-buttermilk pancakes.

1 - cup whole-wheat flour
1 - cup buttermilk
1 - egg
1 - Tbsp vegetable oil
1 - tsp baking powder
½ - tsp baking soda

Stir ingredients until blended. Add ¾ cup blueberries and gently stir. Using medium heat, preheat a non-stick skillet coated with cooking spray. Pour slightly less than ¼ cup of batter onto skillet per pancake. Cook slowly until bubbles break on surface of pancake. Turn and cook until other side is lightly browned. Makes 8 pancakes.

Serves 4. Each pancake is about 95 Calories. Pictured below are wild-blueberry pancakes with two slices of turkey bacon.

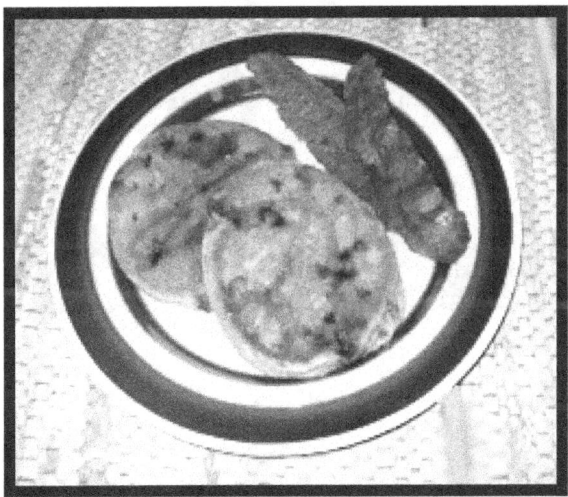

Diet Tip of the Day: A peanut butter sandwich on whole wheat bread with a glass of skim milk and an apple makes a nutritious, reasonably low-calorie lunch.

Day 4 Recipe

London Broil

  1 lb boneless flank steak about ¾" thick, fat trimmed
  1 clove garlic
  1 teaspoon dry oregano

Rub each side of the flank steak with garlic. Season with oregano, salt and pepper to taste. Prepare a large non-stick skillet over high heat. Steak should sizzle when placed on hot skillet. Sear steak on one side for about 5 minutes; then turn and sear other side for about 4 minutes, or until done to preference. Check the center by making small incision. Carve into ¼-inch slices.

Serves 4. About 320 Calories per serving (for meat only).

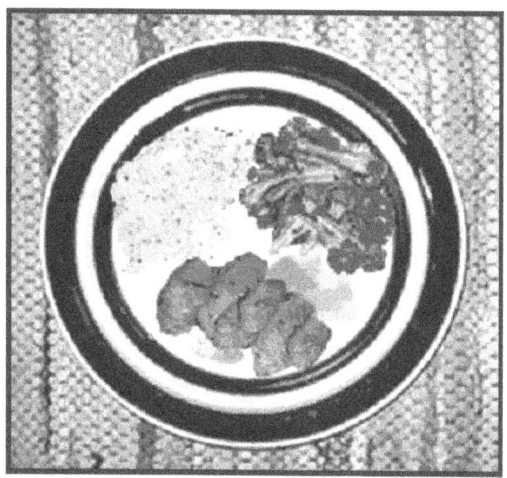

Diet Tip of the Day: Stay Busy. Most people will do anything to avoid work, housework, yard work, exercise, etc. But any kind of work burns a lot more calories than just sitting! Whatever it is you are avoiding – just go do it!

Day 5 Recipe

No recipe today. The **frozen dinner** for Day 5 of the 900-Calorie Diet must contain no more than 220 Calories.

The **frozen dinner** for Day 5 of the 1200-Calorie Diet must contain no more than 300 Calories.

See **Appendix D** (page 45) for a list of available frozen dinners ranging from 160 to 300 Calories.

Understand that in some instances, frozen may actually be better than fresh, because if you keep fresh fruit and vegetables in your fridge for a long time, they lose some of their nutritional value. Whereas, frozen foods are usually processed and packaged within hours of being picked. And the freezing process itself does not destroy nutrients. So buying frozen and then defrosting when you want the fruit or vegetable can actually retain more nutrients.

According to the U.S. Department of Agriculture, food stored continuously at 0 °F is always safe to eat. Freezing keeps food safe and preserves food for extended periods because it prevents the growth of microorganisms that cause food spoilage and illness. **Please read the important Frozen-Food Safety Warning in Appendix E.**

Use an appliance thermometer to monitor your freezer's temperature. If a refrigerator freezing compartment can't maintain 0° F or if the freezer door is opened frequently, use it for short-term food storage, and eat those foods as soon as possible for best quality. Use a free-standing freezer set at 0° F or below for long-term storage of frozen foods. Again, keep a thermometer in your freezing compartment or freezer to check the temperature.

Because freezing keeps food safe almost indefinitely, recommended freezer storage times are to preserve quality (taste, etc) of food, not the safety or nutritional value. **The quality of frozen dinners or entrees in a freezer at 0 °F will be maintained for 3 to 4 months.**

If there is a power outage, or if your freezer fails, or if the freezer door is left ajar by mistake, the food may still be safe to use. As long as a freezer with its door ajar continues to run, to cool, the foods should stay safe overnight. If a repairman is on the way or it appears the power will be restored soon, just keep your freezer door closed. A freezer full of food will usually keep about 2 days if the door is kept shut; a half-full freezer will last about a day. The freezing compartment of a refrigerator may not keep foods frozen as long . If the freezer is not full, group all packages together to help maintain their low temperature.

During a power failure, you may want to put dry ice, a block or bags of ice in the freezer, or transfer foods to a friend's freezer until power returns. Again, use an appliance thermometer to monitor the temperature. To determine the safety of foods when the power goes on, check their condition and temperature. If food is partly frozen, still has ice crystals, or is as cold as if it were in a refrigerator (40 °F), it is safe to refreeze or use. It's not necessary to cook raw foods before refreezing. **If in doubt discard the food. And always discard frozen food whose temperature has exceeded 40 °F for more than two hours.**

<u>Diet Tip of the Day:</u> **Buy a pedometer** and start walking. For the average person 2,100 steps amounts to walking about one mile. A Harvard study has shown that 8,000 to 10,000 step per day promotes weight loss.

Day 6 Recipe

Baked Herb-Crusted Cod

    4 - 4 to 5 ounce cod fish fillets
    2 - tablespoons (Tbsp) flour
    2 - Tbsp cornmeal
    2 - Tbsp minced fresh herbs
    2 - teaspoons (tsp) lemon juice

Sprinkle cod with lemon juice. Mix flour, cornmeal and herbs and dust the cod with the cornmeal- herb mixture. Bake in oven at 375 °F for 10 minutes. Add salt and black pepper to taste.

Serves 4. One serving is about 230 Calories (for cod only).

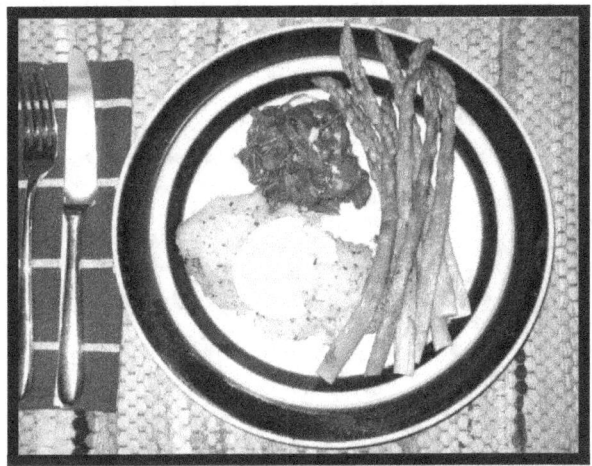

Diet Tip of the Day: **Take a daily multi-vitamin/mineral supplement.** This is important when you're on a diet – as a kind of insurance policy.

Day 7 Recipe

Pasta with Marinara Sauce

Tomato sauce: Sauté ½ small onion, chopped fine, in 1 tsp olive oil. Add two finely chopped garlic cloves, 1½ cups chopped plum tomatoes and ½ tsp chopped fresh oregano. Stir and cook about 5 minutes on a low flame. (Later add about ¼ cup of the pasta liquid to the sauce to thin it.)

    ½ pound <u>whole-wheat</u> pasta

    ¼ tsp salt

Bring 2 quarts of lightly salted water to a boil. Add pasta and stir occasionally (to keep pasta from sticking to the bottom of the pot). Keep water boiling and cook until pasta are "al dente." (Cooking time is approximately 9 minutes.) Drain pasta. (Remember to add some of the pasta liquid to the tomato sauce.). Pour the marinara sauce over the pasta and serve hot.

<u>**Serves 4**</u>. One serving is about 225 Calories.

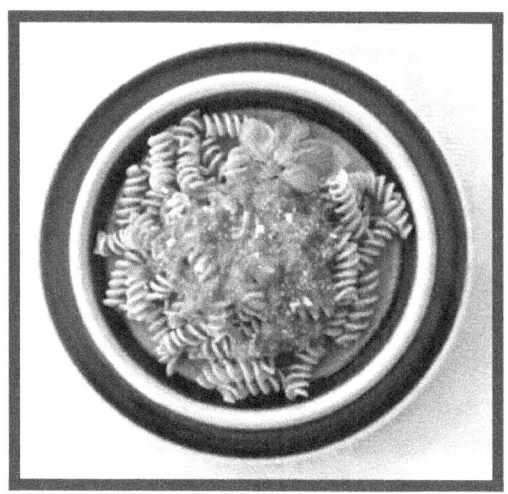

<u>**Diet Tip of the Day:**</u>   **Beware of alcoholic beverages.** Beer has about 13 Calories per ounce, wine 25 Calories per ounce and whiskey 71 Calories per ounce.

Appendix A
Shopping Tips

No cooking doesn't mean no preparation! You will probably have to shop once a week. The following should help you prepare your shopping list.

First, understand that the problem with basing a meal plan on name-brand food items, such as a particular Lean Cuisine frozen entree, is that the item might not be available where you shop, or it may have been discontinued. What to do? That's where Appendices C and D in this eBook come in handy. Appendix C lists 19 name-brand soups in microwaveable bowls. Appendix D lists more than 100 name-brand frozen meals with their calorie count. Using these lists you should be able to find a substitute for the soup or frozen entree you can't find - a substitute that is based on the same food type, e.g., chicken, fish, or meat, and has the same approximate calorie count.

Exchanging Foods

If there is a food listed in the diet you don't like, or perhaps that you forgot to pick up while shopping, you probably can exchange or substitute another food in its place – a technique used by dieticians. Exchanging a food listed in a diet for another food with approximately equal caloric value and nutritional content is the foundation of a successful long-term diet.

Substitution possibilities are almost endless but have to be done carefully. The easiest substitutions are those within the same food group, such as exchanging one vegetable variety for another, or a glass of milk for a cup of yogurt. More sophisticated exchanges cross food groups, for instance replacing 3½ ounces of turkey with a tablespoon of peanut butter spread on a piece of whole wheat bread. Both foods are complete proteins and both contain about 175 Calories. Refer to a good online calorie table to find calorie values. With some understanding and experience, you will be able to substitute foods called for in this diet with equal calorie foods from the same food group.

Another alternative is the following Food Substitution List that suggests substitutions for a variety of food items that appear in the daily meal plans. For example, Day 5 of the diet calls for half a cantaloupe for breakfast. But suppose cantaloupe is not in season, or just doesn't look good, or maybe it's too expensive, or you can't find it at your grocery, from the Food Substitution List you find that you may exchange a ½ cup of orange juice for half cantaloupe – both are in the fruit category and both contain about 50 Calories.

Light Syrup - Use any light syrup (25 Calories per Tbsp)
Big-Bowl Salad - Exchange with unlimited steamed greens (spinach, etc)
Cantaloupe (½) - Use ½ cup Orange juice
Cereal - Exchange with any other whole-grain cereal
Cottage Cheese (1 cup) - Two 8 oz glasses skim milk
Yogurt - Select 6 ounces skim milk
Eggs – Use Egg Beaters
Fresh fruit - ¾ cup canned fruit (no sugar added)
Frozen entrée - Substitute frozen entrée with same calories.
Grapefruit (½) - Choose an orange (medium)
Handful of Nuts - Popcorn Mini Bag
Kashi Chewy Granola Bar - Quaker Chewy Dipps Granola Bar
Kashi Go Lean Waffles - Eggo Nutri-Grain Whole Wheat Frozen Waffles
Hot Pockets Wraps - Lean Pockets Wrap
Morningstar Breakfast Sausage - Any breakfast sausage with comparable calories
String Cheese - Laughing Cow light cheese (2 wedges)
Popcorn - Use handful of mixed nuts
Raisin bread - Plain whole-grain bread
Skinny Cow Ice Cream Sandwich - Skinny Cow Low Fat Fudge Bar
Soup - Choose any soup with same calorie count
Whole-grain Bread - Vary bread type (whole wheat, rye, etc)
Wine (4 oz) - Instead select grapes (1 cup)

Appendix B
Eating Smart

Guidelines for Healthy Eating

No single food can supply all the nutrients you need in the amounts you need. The most important factors in nutrition are variety, variety, variety! **Variety is the key to a nutritious diet.** As a means of setting strategies for food selection, the U.S. Department of Health and Human Services and the Department of Agriculture issue Dietary Guidelines every five years. The 2005 Dietary Guidelines describe a healthy diet as one that:

- Emphasizes fruits, vegetables, whole grains, and fat-free or low-fat milk products.
- Includes fish, poultry, lean meats, beans & nuts.
- Is low in saturated fats, trans fats, cholesterol, salt (sodium) and added sugars.

The guidelines encourage adults to consume a variety of nutrient-dense foods and beverages within their caloric needs. In 2005, the afore mentioned U.S. government agencies recommended how much should be eaten from each of the basic food groups (i.e., from the fruit group, vegetable group, grains group, meat and beans group, milk group, and oils group) to meet your caloric goal – whether you are trying to lose weight or maintain weight. All this information and more can be found in my eBook *Eat Smart for Better Health - U.S. Edition* published by NoPaperPress.

Even though most adults can get all the vitamins and minerals they need by merely consuming a variety of nutritious foods (from the fruit group, the vegetable group, the grains group, the meat and beans group, the milk group, and the oils group), many physicians recommend a daily multi-vitamin mineral supplement – just in case you don't eat the way you should.

Be aware that some micronutrients, such as the fat-soluble vitamin A, can be harmful if taken in large quantities. To be safe your multi-vitamin/mineral supplement should contain no more than 100 percent of the recommended dietary allowance (RDA) for each vitamin or mineral. Generally, you don't need the high doses in multi-vitamin/mineral supplements labeled "therapeutic" or "extra-strength." There may be medical reasons for taking larger amounts of a vitamin or mineral than the RDA provides, but check with your doctor first. For example, a physician may advise a pregnant woman to take an iron supplement, and women who could become pregnant to take folic acid in addition to consuming folate-rich foods to reduce the risk of some serious birth defects. Adults over age 50 and vegetarians who do not eat animal foods may be advised to get their vitamin B_{12} from a supplement or from fortified foods. People with limited exposure to sunlight may need a vitamin D supplement, and individuals who seldom eat dairy products or other rich sources of calcium may need to take a calcium supplement.

As you age, adequate protein intake and body protein reserves are more important than ever, especially during times of emotional and physical stress. Body proteins are constantly being made and used during your lifetime to maintain the functions of the cells and organs, and protein is needed to help to prevent muscle loss. Good sources of protein-rich foods are meats, fish, eggs, dairy products, dried beans and peas, and soy products. Vitamin B_{12} can be a problem nutrient for older adults. Vitamin B_{12} enables your body to manufacture healthy red-blood cells and assists in the transmission of electrical signals between nerve cells. The acid in your stomach helps release vitamin B_{12} from the protein in the food you eat. This must occur before vitamin B_{12} is absorbed in your intestines. But as you age, the amount of stomach acid you produce decreases. Less hydrochloric acid lessens the amount of vitamin B_{12} separated from proteins in foods and can result in poor absorption of vitamin B_{12}. Vitamin B_{12} is found naturally in meat, fish, poultry, eggs and fortified cereals. But recent studies have revealed that up to 30 percent of adults aged 50 years and older may also have atrophic gastritis, an increased growth of intestinal bacteria that renders them unable to normally absorb vitamin B_{12} in food. They are, however, able to absorb the synthetic vitamin B_{12} added to fortified foods and dietary supplements. As a result, fortified foods and vitamin supplements may be the best sources of vitamin B_{12} for adults 50 years and older.

What Makes for a Good Diet?

Every good weight-loss diet must have the following three characteristics: **First**, a good diet must provide you with an understanding of weight control as well as the knowledge you need to reduce your weight to the desired level. **Second**, a good diet must help you remain healthy while you are losing weight. **Third**, a good diet must lead you to a healthier way of eating and exercising that will, in the long term, help you keep off the weight you have lost.

The weight-loss diet featured in this eBook is the so-called "balanced diet;" i.e., a diet that is not only low calorie and reasonably low in fat, but is also nutritionally balanced. The *7-Day Diet for Women*, however, does not meet all the criteria set forth above. While you will get some "dieting insight" and some idea of how much you can eat and still lose weight, you will not get a real understanding of weight control from this eBook. That's not its purpose. What you will get is a healthy diet – and a diet that if followed will promote weight loss. Think of the 7-*Day Diet* as a quick fix, a healthy start that will get you on the right track – but it's not the long-term answer.

Long-term success is about developing both an understanding and a plan that will result in healthier eating and physical activity habits. The desire to lose weight and the discipline to start and stay on a weight-control program are crucial. But along with desire and discipline, it is our belief that **only an in-depth understanding of weight control, nutrition and exercise will lead to long-term success**. For a through understanding and the guidance you need to succeed in the long term I recommend you read, *Weight Control - U.S. Edition* by Vincent Antonetti, Ph.D., an eBook also published by NoPaperPress.

Breakfast Guidelines

You've heard it before. It's important to start the day right and eat breakfast. **So try to allow time for breakfast before you rush off to work.** If need be do some preliminary preparation the night before such as setting up your coffee maker, deciding on and measuring the amount of cereal you will be eating, etc. Many busy people prepare breakfast at home and bring it to work in a plastic container. Do what you need to do – but don't skip breakfast!

In the 7-*Day Diet,* you may substitute wholesome **whole-grain cereal** for any specified cereal. For example, if you're not crazy about having Shredded Wheat for breakfast on Day 6, substitute Wheat Chex or Cheerios, etc. And if you don't like the fried egg called for on Day 5, have a hard-boiled egg or make a scrambled egg instead. Maybe the cantaloupe called for in the meal plan is not in season. No problem. Just replace the cantaloupe with a half cup of orange juice. Find a more complete list of food substitutions and exchanges go to Appendix A (page 33).

Lunch Guidelines

On most days of the *7-Day Diet for Women,* lunch will call for either soup or a sandwich. Feel free to substitute a soup you favor in place of those indicated – provided the basic type of soup and calorie counts are similar to those specified in the *7-Day Diet for Women.* For example, Day 1 calls for a cup of Lentil Soup (140 Calories), but if you prefer, you may substitute a cup of Navy Bean Soup – which is in the same food group as lentil soup and contains approximately the same calorie count.

Warm Weather Substitutions: On warm and especially very hot days, you may want to substitute a sandwich, a tuna or salmon salad for the soup of the day.

Dinner Guidelines

On the *7-Day Diet for Women*, one of the dinner mainstays is a "Tossed Green Salad." Prepare your "Tossed Green Salad" in a bowl with a volume of at least 16 ounces, or 2 cups. First add about 1 cup of either green leaf lettuce, Romaine lettuce or a mesclun mix. Then add, as desired, half cup of green veggies such as broccoli, celery, cucumber, peppers, spinach, or watercress. This vegetable combination will, on average, total about 35 Calories. You will be eating a "Tossed Green Salad" just about every day at dinnertime. Remember that variety is the key to a nutritious diet. So be sure to vary the ingredients of the salad.

Top your "Tossed Green Salad" with 2 tablespoons of any light salad dressing available at your local supermarket that contains no more than 20 to 25 Calories per tablespoon. Some of my favorite light salad dressings are:
- **Ken's Steakhouse Fat Free Raspberry Pecan**
- **Kraft Light Done Right House Italian**
- **Wishbone Just 2 Good Honey Dijon**
- **Newman's Lighten Up! Balsamic Vinaigrette**

Your "Tossed Green Salad" with salad dressing will cost you roughly 70 Calories but will be packed with lots of health-giving vitamins, minerals and fiber.

Snack Guidelines

On some of the menus in the *7-Day Diet for Women* feature a morning snack, an afternoon snack and an evening snack. The main snacks are:

Yogurt: I recommend Dannon Light at 90 Calories per container (at this writing). Select any flavor. There are other brands you may prefer but whatever you buy be certain you eat no more than 90 Calories worth of yogurt for your snack.

Fresh Fruit in season: Choose an apple, pear, peach, plum, watermelon (1 cup), etc. You will be eating fruit every day. So vary the fruit that you select to get good array of micronutrients.

Handful of Unsalted Mixed Nuts: Nuts and seeds are loaded with protein and fiber. This eBook uses a "handful" as a convenient descriptor rather than something like "16 almonds = 100 Calories," but be aware that although nuts are a healthy food, nuts are also a high-calorie food. Buy mixed nuts to get a range of micronutrients. And please no salt.

Skinny Cow Ice Cream Sandwich: This is a relatively low-calorie, low fat, yummy dairy-sweet snack.

Kashi TLC Chewy Granola Bar: A sweet treat packed with whole grains, nuts and seeds. The bar comes in four flavors – with each containing about 140 Calories.

Popcorn: Popcorn is a tasty, nutritious high-fiber, filling snack. A Popcorn Mini Bag, such as Orville Redenbacher's Smart Pop is convenient and contains 110 Calories. But for the best popcorn I suggest you purchase a hot-air popper which uses popping corn, a type of corn that bursts from the kernel and puffs up when heated. A hot-air popper will make a large batch of popcorn in a few minutes. For a snack, eat only 5 or 6 cups of the popcorn and store the remainder for another day. At this writing, you can buy a hot-air popper for approximately $25.00.

About Bread

First understand that bread, more specifically whole-grain breads, are good sources of complex carbohydrates and dietary fiber, as well as several B vitamins (thiamin, riboflavin, niacin, and folate), vitamin E, and minerals (iron, magnesium and selenium).

In recent years, however, sliced bread loaves have gotten larger, as have the bread slices inside these loaves. Just a few years ago the standard slice of bread contained about 70 Calories – now most are 100 plus Calories.

The *7-Day Diet* **requires whole-grain bread at 70 Calories per slice.** Quite a few bakers sell thin sliced or "light" sliced bread. The difficult part is finding a whole grain thin sliced or "light" bread (with about 70 Calories per slice). Whatever the brand, make sure the first word in the Ingredients list is "whole." "Pepperidge Farm Small Slice 100% Whole Wheat" is a good choice. It's whole grain, has 70 Calories per slice and it tastes good too.

Important Notes

1) Coffee or tea may be decaf or regular. If desired, skim milk and a sugar substitute may be added to coffee or tea. And soy or almond milk may be used instead of cow's milk.

2) Fried eggs, scrambled eggs, or an omelet should be cooked in a pan coated with a non-stick cooking spray.

3) On bread, corn on the cob and baked potatoes, if desired, you may use a zero-calorie butter substitute spray. Do not use butter!

4) Cereals should be whole grain and preferably without added sugar. At the top of the list are Old-fashioned Oat Meal, Wheatena and Shredded Wheat. Among other reasonably healthy choices are Cheerios, Wheat Chex, Wheaties, some Kashi cereals and Farina.

5) Bread may be either plain or toasted whole grain, such as whole wheat, whole rye or pumpernickel. If desired, bread may be sprayed with a zero-calorie butter substitute.

6) Use only lean cuts of meat trimmed of all visible fat. Poultry should be limited to chicken or turkey breasts (white meat only and skinless). Make sure the turkey bacon you use contains no more than 35 Calories per slice.

7) When canned tuna or salmon is specified, use only fish packed in water.

8) An unlimited amount of green salad may be eaten, but the salad dressing should be as specified.

9) Use freely as desired: clear unsweetened coffee, clear unsweetened tea, water, seltzer, any diet soda, clear soups without fat, bouillon, and seasonings such as mustard, cinnamon, dill, herbs, red and black pepper, curry, vinegar, lemon juice and sections, and dill and sour pickles.

10) Any specified snack may be moved to any other part of the day, and/or combined with breakfast, lunch or dinner.

Keeping It Of

Within five years, more than 90 percent of all dieters regain every pound they have lost. Why? In most cases it's because after losing weight most people eventually revert to their pre-diet eating and exercising habits, and this inevitably leads to their regaining the weight they lost– and often more. The fact is the less you weigh, the less you need to eat to sustain your lower weight.

A study, published in the Annals of Internal Medicine, that followed 4,000 people for three decades suggests that in the long term, 90 percent of men and 70 percent of women will become overweight. Interestingly, half of the men and women in the study, who had made it well into adulthood without a weight problem, ultimately also became overweight and a third actually became obese. The point being that you can never become complacent. You must continually watch your weight because we are all at risk of becoming overweight.

As mentioned previously, the key to long-term weight control success is knowledge and understanding, combined of course with desire and self-discipline. I suggest you read *Weight Maintenance - U.S. Edition* by Vincent Antonetti, Ph.D. (also published by NoPaperPress) – absolutely the best weight maintenance book on the market.

Appendix C
Soup Selections

When the Daily Meal Plan menu specifies soup have only one serving (8 ounces) unless stated otherwise. Note that the listed soups were available in most supermarkets as of 07/24/2020. *These are canned soup selections.

Soup Description	Calories
Healthy Choice Chicken with Rice	90
Campbell's Tomato	100
Healthy Choice Country Vegetable	100
Progresso Minestrone*	110
Progresso Chickarina*	110
Progresso Italian-Style Wedding*	120
Campbell's Home-Style Light Chicken Corn Chowder*	120
Campbell's Home-Style Chicken Noodle	130
Campbell's Home-Style Butter Nut Squash*	130
Campbell's Healthy Request Vegetable Beef	140
Progresso Lentil*	140
Progresso Green Split Pea*	150
Campbell's Slow Kettle New England Clam Chowder	160
Progresso Macaroni and Bean*	160
Progresso New England Clam Chowder*	170
Progresso Lasagna-Style*	170
Progresso Broccoli Cheese with Bacon*	180
Also may have 2 servings of a 90 Calorie soup	180
Campbell's Chunky Classic Chicken Noodle	190
Amy's Rustic Italian Vegetable*	190
Campbell's Chunky Beef n Cheese*	200
Amy's French Country Vegetable*	210
Campbell's Chunky Sirloin Burger + Vegetables	220
Enjoy two servings of a 110 or 120 Calorie soup	230
Enjoy two servings of a 120 Calorie soup	240

Appendix D
Frozen Dinner Entrees

Appendix D lists three popular brands of frozen entrées: Healthy Choice, Lean Cuisine and Smart Ones. The listing is further divided by entrée type: Poultry entrées, Meat entrées, Seafood entrées, Pasta entrées, Pizza and Other entrées. The entire table is arranged from the lowest to highest in calories. Note that the listed frozen entrées were available in most super markets as of 07/24/2020.

Entrée Type	Name	Brand	Calories
Poultry	Tomato Basil Chicken & Spinach	Smart Ones	160
Poultry	Chicken Santa Fe	Smart Ones	160
Meat	Asian Style Beef & Broccoli	Smart Ones	160
Meat	Steak Portobella	Lean Cuisine	160
Seafood	Shrimp Alfredo	Lean Cuisine	160
Poultry	Herb Roasted Chicken	Lean Cuisine	170
Poultry	Chipotle Lime Chicken	Smart Ones	170
Poultry	Grilled Chicken Marsala	Healthy Choice	180
Poultry	Creamy Basil Chicken & Broccoli	Smart Ones	180
Poultry	Pomegranate Chicken	Lean Cuisine	180
Meat	Sweet Siracha Braised Beef	Lean Cuisine	180
Meat	Beef Merlot	Healthy Choice	180
Meat	Homestyle Beef Pot Roast	Smart Ones	180
Poultry	Roasted Turkey & Vegetables	Lean Cuisine	190
Poultry	Chicken & Broccoli Alfredo	Healthy Choice	190
Poultry	Chicken & Vegetable Stir Fry	Healthy Choice	190
Other	Broccoli & Cheddar Roast Potato	Smart Ones	190
Poultry	Home Style Chicken & Potatoes	Healthy Choice	200
Poultry	Crustless Chicken Pot Pie	Smart Ones	200
Poultry	Cheddar Bacon Chicken	Lean Cuisine	200
Pasta	Pasta Primavera	Smart Ones	200
Poultry	Slow Roasted Turkey Breast	Smart Ones	210

Poultry	Lemon Herb Chicken Piccata	Smart Ones	210
Poultry	Honey Balsamic Chicken	Healthy Choice	210
Pasta	Ravioli Florentine	Smart Ones	210
Poultry	Cajun Style Chicken & Shrimp	Healthy Choice	220
Poultry	Chicken Margherita	Smart Ones	220
Meat	Roast Beef & Mashed Potatoes	Smart Ones	220
Pasta	Creamy Pasta Romano	Smart Ones	220
Meat	Roast Beef & Mashed Potatoes	Smart Ones	220
Meat	Meat Loaf with Mashed Potatoes	Lean Cuisine	230
Meat	Pulled Pork & Black Beans	Smart Ones	230
Seafood	Shrimp & Angel Hair Pasta	Lean Cuisine	230
Pasta	Cheese Ravioli Mushroom Sauce	Smart Ones	230
Poultry	Chicken Carbonara	Lean Cuisine	240
Poultry	Creamy Basil Chick & Tortenllini	Lean Cuisine	240
Poultry	Glazed Chicken	Lean Cuisine	240
Poultry	Honey Glazed Turkey & Potatoes	Healthy Choice	240
Pasta	Spicy Penne Arrabbiata	Lean Cuisine	240
Pasta	Cheese Ravioli	Lean Cuisine	250
Pasta	Vermont Cheddar Mac & Cheese	Lean Cuisine	250
Pasta	Fettuccini Alfredo	Smart Ones	250
Pasta	Lasagna Bake with Meat Sauce	Smart Ones	250
Poultry	Fiesta Grilled Chicken	Lean Cuisine	250
Poultry	Baked Chicken	Lean Cuisine	250
Pasta	Chicken Linguini Red Pepper	Healthy Choice	250
Poultry	Golden Roasted Turkey Breast	Healthy Choice	250
Poultry	Chicken Mesquite	Smart Ones	250
Poultry	Chicken Oriental	Smart Ones	250
Poultry	Orange Sesame Chicken	Smart Ones	250
Poultry	Teriyaki Chicken & Vegetables	Smart Ones	250
Seafood	Tuna Noodle Casserole	Smart Ones	250

Poultry	Grilled Chicken Primavera	Lean Cuisine	260
Poultry	Chicken & Noodles	Healthy Choice	260
Meat	Barbecue Steak w Red Potatoes	Healthy Choice	260
Pasta	Tortellini Primavera Parmesan	Healthy Choice	260
Pasta	Sesame Noodles with Vegetables	Smart Ones	260
Pasta	Creamy Rigatoni w Chicken	Smart Ones	260
Pasta	Macaroni & Cheese	Smart Ones	260
Pasta	Butternut Squash Ravioli	Lean Cuisine	260
Other	Santa Fe Rice & Beans	Smart Ones	260
Other	Coconut Chickpea Curry	Lean Cuisine	260
Poultry	Glazed Turkey Tenderloins	Lean Cuisine	270
Poultry	Kung Pao Chicken	Healthy Choice	270
Poultry	Chicken Margherita w Balsamic	Healthy Choice	270
Poultry	Chicken Strips & Sweet Potatoes	Smart Ones	270
Poultry	Thai Style Chicken Rice Noodle	Smart Ones	270
Meat	Salisbury Steak with Mac & Cheese	Lean Cuisine	270
Meat	Sweet & Spicy Harissa Meatballs	Lean Cuisine	270
Meat	Meat Loaf	Smart Ones	270
Pasta	Classic Macaroni & Beef	Lean Cuisine	270
Pasta	Mushroom Mezzaluna Ravioli	Lean Cuisine	270
Other	Vegetable Fried Rice	Smart Ones	280
Other	Asian Pot Stickers	Lean Cuisine	280
Poultry	Sesame Stir Fry with Chicken	Lean Cuisine	280
Poultry	Chicken in Sweet BBQ Sauce	Lean Cuisine	280
Poultry	Apple Cranberry Chicken	Lean Cuisine	280
Poultry	Chicken Fettuccini Alfredo	Healthy Choice	280
Poultry	Grilled Chicken Marinara	Healthy Choice	280
Poultry	Sweet & Spicy Orange Chicken	Healthy Choice	280
Poultry	Chicken Parmesan	Smart Ones	280
Poultry	Turkey Breast with Stuffing	Smart Ones	280

Meat	Beef & Broccoli	Healthy Choice	280
Meat	Meatball Marinara	Healthy Choice	280
Meat	Beef Teriyaki	Healthy Choice	280
Pasta	Spinach Artichoke Ravioli	Lean Cuisine	280
Pasta	Alfredo Pasta w Chicken & Broc	Lean Cuisine	280
Pasta	Three Cheese Ziti Marinara	Smart Ones	280
Pasta	Spinach Artichoke Ravioli	Lean Cuisine	280
Pasta	Alfredo Pasta w Chicken & Broccol	Lean Cuisine	280
Pasta	Linguini with Ricotta & Spinach	Lean Cuisine	280
Pasta	Spaghetti & Meatballs	Healthy Choice	280
Pasta	Spaghetti with Meat Sauce	Smart Ones	280
Other	Vegetable Fried Rice	Smart Ones	280
Other	Asian Pot Stickers	Lean Cuisine	280
Poultry	Chicken with Almonds	Lean Cuisine	290
Poultry	Chicken with Peanut Sauce	Lean Cuisine	290
Poultry	Chicken Fettuccini	Lean Cuisine	290
Poultry	Grilled Chicken Pesto w Veggies	Healthy Choice	290
Poultry	General Tso's Spicy Chicken	Healthy Choice	290
Poultry	Pineapple Chicken	Healthy Choice	290
Poultry	Chicken Enchiladas Suiza	Smart Ones	290
Meat	Swedish Meatballs	Lean Cuisine	290
Seafood	Parmesan Crusted Fish	Lean Cuisine	290
Seafood	Lemon Pepper Fish	Healthy Choice	290
Pasta	Pasta with Swedish Meatballs	Smart Ones	290
Pasta	Pasta with Ricotta & Spinach	Smart Ones	290
Pizza	Thin Crust Cheese Pizza	Smart Ones	290
Other	Cheese & Bean Enchilada	Lean Cuisine	290
Poultry	Sweet & Sour Chicken	Lean Cuisine	300
Poultry	Chicken Fried Rice	Lean Cuisine	300
Poultry	Crustless Chicken Pot Pie	Healthy Choice	300

NoPaperPress Paperbacks and eBooks

100-Day Super Diet-1200 Calorie*
100-Day Super Diet-1500 Calorie*
100-Day No-Cooking Diet-1200 Cal*
100-Day No-Cooking Diet-1500 Cal*
90-Day Smart Diet-1200 Calorie*
90-Day Smart Diet-1500 Calorie*
90-Day No-Cooking Diet - 1200 Cal*
90-Day No-Cooking Diet - 1500 Cal*
90-Day Perfect Diet - 1200 Calorie*
90-Day Perfect Diet - 1500 Calorie*
60-Day Perfect Diet-1200 Calorie*
60-Day Perfect Diet-1500 Calorie*
50-Day Flex Diet-1200 Calorie*
50-Day Flex Diet-1500 Calorie*
30-Day Quick Diet - for Women*
30-Day Quick Diet - for Men*
30-Day No-Cooking Diet*
30-Day Diet for Women - Metric*
25 Day Easy Diet-1200 Calorie*
25 Day Easy Diet-1500 Calorie*
25-Day No-Cooking Diet
10-Day Express Diet
10-Day No-Cooking Diet*
7-Day Diet for Women*
7-Day Diet for Men*
7-Day No-Cooking Diets*
90-Day Gluten-Free Diet-1200 Cal*
90-Day Gluten-Free Diet-1500 Cal*
30-Day Gluten-Free Quick Diet*
30-Day Gluten-Free No-Cooking Diet*
7-Day Diet for Women - Metric*
7-Day Diet for Men - Metric
7-Day Gluten-Free Express Diet*
7-Day Gluten-Free No-Cooking Diet*
90-Day Vegetarian Diet-1200 Calorie*
90-Day Vegetarian Diet-1500 Calorie*
30-Day Vegetarian Diet*
7-Day Vegetarian Diet*
Weight Loss for Women*
Weight Loss for Women - Metric
Weight Loss for Women - UK
Weight Loss for Men*
Maximum Weight Loss - 1200 Cal*
Maximum Weight Loss - 1500 Cal*

Weight Loss for Men - Metric*
Maximum Weight Loss- 1200 Calorie*
Maximum Weight Loss- 1500 Calorie*
Weight Control - U.S. Edition
Weight Control - Metric. Edition
Professional Weight Control Women - U.S.
Professional Weight Control Women - Metric
Professional Weight Control Men - U.S.
Professional Weight Control Men - Metric
Weight Maintenance - U.S. Edition*
Weight Maintenance - Metric. Edition*
Weight Maintenance - UK Edition
Weight Loss for Senior Men*
Weight Loss for Senior Women*
Eat Smart - U.S. Edition*
Eat Smart - Metric Edition
30-Day Mediterranean Diet
Exercise Smart - U.S. Edition*
Exercise Smart - UK Edition*
Total Fitness - U.S. Edition
Total Fitness - Metric Edition
Total Fitness - UK Edition
Total Fitness for Women-U.S. Edition*
Total Fitness for Women - Metric
Total Fitness for Women - UK Edition
Total Fitness for Men - U.S. Edition*
Total Fitness for Men- Metric Edition*
Total Fitness for Men - UK Edition
Senior Fitness - U.S. Edition*
Senior Fitness - Metric Edition*
Senior Fitness - UK Edition*
Computer Diet - U.S. Edition*
Computer Diet - Metric Edition*
Reliable Weight Loss - U.S. Edition
101 Weight Loss Tips*
101 Healthy Eating Tips*
101 Lifelong Fitness Tips*
101 Weight Maintenance Tips
101 Weight Loss Recipes
101 Gluten-Free Weight Loss Recipes
101 Vegetarian Weight Loss Recipes*
30-Day Mediterranean Diet*
90-Day Mediterranean Diet - 1200 Cal*
90-Day Mediterranean Diet - 1500 Cal*

* These titles are available as both ebooks and paperbacks. The ebooks are sold by Amazon, Apple, Google, Barnes & Noble and Kobo. Our paperbacks are only sold by Amazon.

Disclaimer

This ebook offers general meal planning, nutrition and weight control information. It is not a medical manual and the author does not claim to be medically qualified. The material in this book is not intended to be a substitute for medical counseling. Everyone should have a medical checkup before beginning a weight loss program. Moreover, the physician conducting the medical exam should be made aware of and should approve the specific weight control program planned. Additionally, while the author and publisher have made every effort to ensure the accuracy of the information in this book, they make no representations or warranties regarding its accuracy or completeness . Further, neither the author nor publisher assume liability for any medical problems that might result from applying the methods in this book, or for any loss of profit, or any other commercial damages, including but not limited to special, incidental, consequential or other damages, and any such liability is hereby expressly disclaimed.